Kids Constipation Cure

Cure it Fast Naturally

by Doria Jones

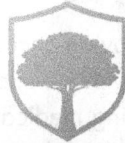

CLADD
PUBLISHING

Cladd Publishing Inc.
USA

This publication is designed to provide accurate information regarding the
subject matter covered. It is sold with the understanding that neither the
author nor the publisher is providing medical, legal or other professional
advice or services. Always seek advice from a competent professional
before using any of the information in this book. The author and the
publisher specifically disclaim any liability that is incurred from the use or
application of the contents of this book.

Kids Constipation Cure: Cure it Fast Naturally

ISBN 978-1-946881-69-4 (e-book)
ISBN 978-1-946881-68-7 (paperback)

Contents

Introduction

Unfortunately, chronic constipation is a very common problem among kids. A child is considered constipated when they have fewer than seven bowel movements in a week; has trouble having a bowel movement; or when the poo is hard and dry.

A child suffering from chronic or the onset of constipation should be treated seriously.

A bowel movement is our bodies natural mechanism for removing things that we don't need like, toxins, heavy metals, medication residue, sugars, parasites and candida.

However, constipation is not something to be embarrassed about. And if your child has been suffering from it, then you understand it's downright debilitating. Before running to the doctors for a laxative or medication, relieve their discomfort fast, and cure it forever with these 41 easy tricks.

Signs of Constipation

Keep in mind that different kids have different bathroom habits. One child might go less, but three times a day; while another might go more, but only once a day.

SIGNS OF CONSTIPATION IN KIDS INCLUDE:
- going less than once daily
- having trouble or pain when going to the bathroom
- feeling full or bloated
- experiencing terrible gas pains
- straining to poop
- seeing a little blood on the toilet paper

It's also common for kids with constipation to sometimes stain their underwear.

Common Causes of Constipation

10 COMMON CAUSES:

1. Constipation usually is due to a diet that doesn't include enough water and fiber, which help the bowels move properly.

2. Lack of routine for drinking, eating, using the restroom and bed.

3. Kids who eat nothing but processed foods.

4. Eating too much dairy products.

5. Sometimes, medicines like antidepressants and those used to treat iron deficiencies cause constipation.

6. Constipation can happen in babies as they change from breast milk to baby formula, or from baby food to solid food.

7. Toddlers who are toilet training can become constipated because they are nervous to go.

8. Some kids avoid going to the bathroom because they don't want to stop playing a fun game, or ask an adult to be excused to go to the bathroom. Ignoring the urge to go makes it harder to go later.

9. Kids can get constipated when they're anxious about something, like starting at a new school or problems at home.

10. Your child is suffering from a lack of good gut flora. This is sometimes caused by vaccinations, antibiotics, poor diet, lack of hydration and chemicals found in food and water supplies.

Toxic Build-up

The average child has 5-10 pounds of poo trapped in their digestive system. The poo is rotting away in the small and large intestines, causing a plethora of bacteria and parasites to flourish!

As the toxic poo builds up, their body becomes weakened. they will start to feel the sickness that constipation causes like, fatigue, weight gain, digestive issues, leaky gut syndrome, constipation, diarrhea, eczema, psoriasis, rosacea, acne, brain fog, attention issues, mood swings, anxiety and depression and much more.

COMMON HEALTH RELATED ISSUES:

- Childhood obesity
- Extreme gas pains
- Type 2 diabetes
- Insomnia
- Mood swings and fits
- Depression
- Inflammation
- Joint pain
- Heart disease
- Memory loss
- Low attention span
- Tiredness
- And much, much more!

It may come as a shock, but our digestive system houses over 80% of the bodies entire immune system. If your child is not producing well-formed stools, then they are suffering from a toxic build up inside their digestive system.

14 Crazy Facts About the Gut

1. Most people have up to 8 undigested meals in their gut at any given time.

2. The gut is home to 80% of your immune system.

3. A healthy gut consists of mostly good bacteria and a small amount of bad bacteria. The good-bad bacteria are known as the gut flora.

4. It is believed that an ideal ratio of good-to-bad gut flora is 85:15.

5. Antibiotics kill our good gut flora.

6. Antibiotics get into our food through meats and dairy products. Unless organic or otherwise stated, farm animals are fed antibiotics. They consume over 55% of all the antibiotics used. Therefore, the EU has banned importing meats raised this way.

7. Fast-growing Candida is the number one bad bacteria in our gut. When the gut is out of balance it can overgrow and cause Candidiasis. This causes swelling and inflammation in the gut. Thus, allows more food particles to pass through the lining

without proper digestion. This is also known as leaky gut.

8.   Once Candida is left unchecked it can have thousands of roots, some as long as 3 feet, that grow into surrounding tissue. This causes intense inflammation and tissue destruction in joints, muscles, gut, and the brain.

9.   A Candida cell wall has the same amino acid sequence as gluten. This can be very confusing to people who are testing negative on a gluten test, but have severe reactions to gluten.

10.   Chlorine and fluoride, commonly found in tap water, also kills good gut bacteria.

11.   Stress can cause the gut to become unbalanced. Our gut releases the hormone Cortisol in stressful situations, which depresses the immune system and raises blood sugar levels. This creates a perfect environment for Candida growth.

12.   Our gut has its own nervous system called, the Enteric Nervous System. This has more neurons than the spinal system and produces 90% of the body's serotonin. Serotonin controls our sense of well-being and happiness. In addition, 50% of our

body's dopamine is also created in the gut. This gives us our sense of reward & pleasure.

A Balanced Gut = A Properly Pooping Butt

When your child's gut is balanced, their body is working at full capacity. When it is not, the digestive system becomes impaired and their health rapidly deteriorates.

NUTRIENT DEPRIVED

All of your vitamin, mineral and nutrient absorption is handled through the digestive process. The body's source of nutrition comes from the foods they eat. However, if their body lacks the ability to efficiently absorb the vital nutrients it needs, they will get sick! If their gut is unbalanced or burdened with toxic waste, your child's ability to absorb becomes impaired, leading to malnutrition, deficiencies, and illness!

PROTECTION FROM INFECTION & ILLNESS

80% of our immune system is housed in the digestive system! In addition to digestion and absorption of necessary nutrients from our food, it is responsible for fighting diseases, infections and illnesses. If you find your child getting sick more than normal, this is a tell-tale sign that their digestive system and immune system are struggling.

SLOW METABOLISM

- Are they suffering from a slow metabolism?

- Gaining weight for no apparent reason?
- **This is all your gut's fault!**

Our metabolism is regulated by our gut. Studies have shown that the bacteria living in the digestive system are directly related to weight management and metabolism. When they are backed up and filled with bad bacteria, their weight will soar.

MOOD AND LEVEL OF HAPPINESS

There is a direct link between an unhealthy gut and mood swings, anxiety, depression and unhappiness! An unbalanced gut filled with garbage causes us to be tired, stressed, increased anxiety, and even depressed.

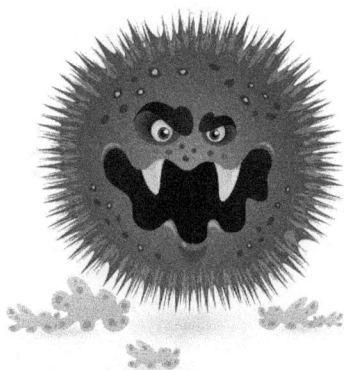

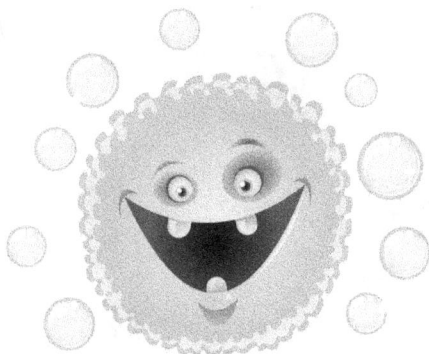

1: Your Gut Flora Is Like a Pond of Fish

Our gut flora "good/bad" bacteria is much like a pond full of fish. The gut is the pond, and the flora is the types of fish that are swimming around. You obviously want to have an abundant of good fish that keep you at your optimal health.

However, these two types of fish have different diets. The good fish thrive on raw fruits, vegetables, beans, seeds, nuts etc. While the bad fish eat sugars, and enjoy breeding in an acidic environment.

By now I am sure that you are realizing that your child has been feeding their bad bacteria and starving their good ones. It doesn't take too long before their 85:15 ratio is out of balance.

2: Probiotics

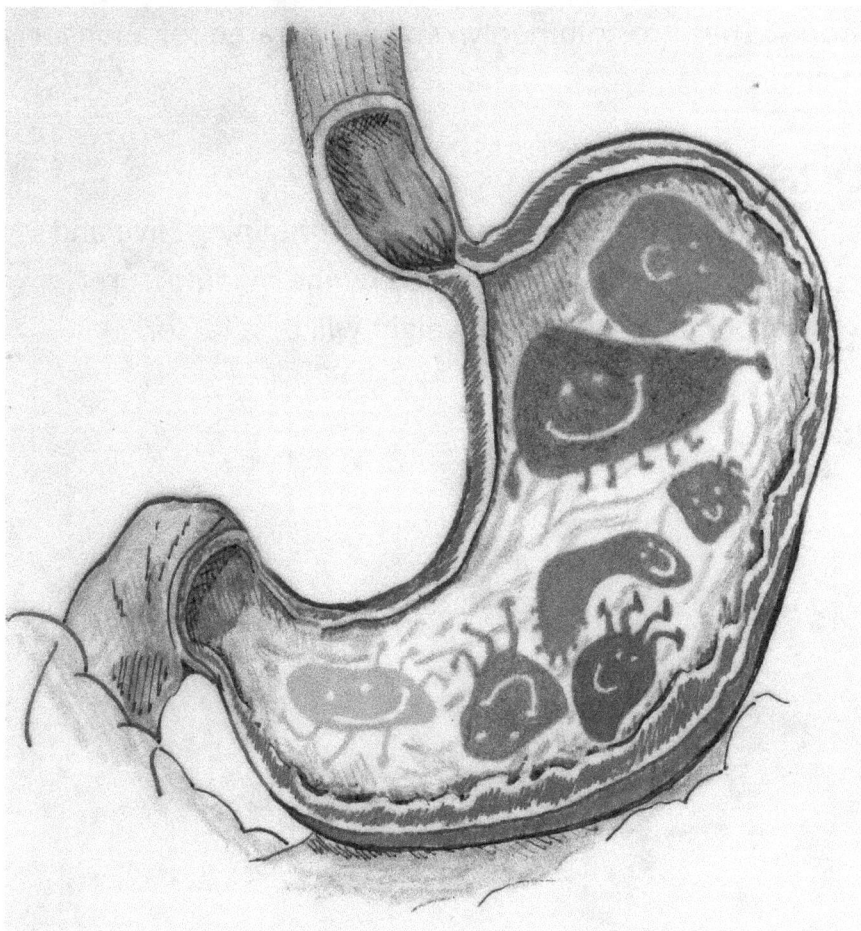

Probiotics is a key element in creating a healthy intestinal tract. It will replenish your good gut bacteria, which allows your body to properly digest food.

When you have a proper ratio of gut flora 85:15 their health will be running at optimal levels. If they have recently taken an antibiotic, be sure to increase their probiotic intake for several weeks to rectify the damage.

Probiotics can be found in the health food section of most stores. They are commonly kept refrigerated for a longer shelf life.

DIRECTIONS

- Take a probiotic supplement containing "live and active" daily as prescribed by the manufacturer. Your child's age and weight will be a factor.

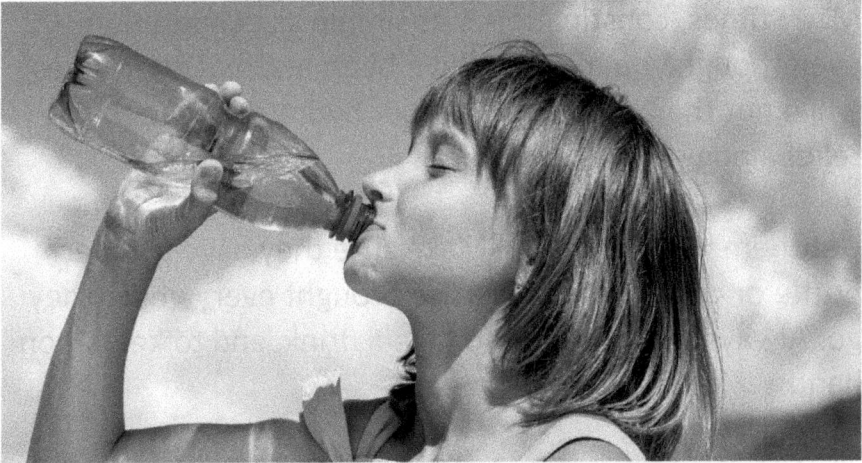

3: Dehydration Is a Killer

For your child's gut to function properly they will need lots of clean water. Your body is incredible at regulating water, if it gets the amount it needs. If it doesn't get enough, your body will withhold as much water as it can to maintain important bodily functions like blood, brain and organ health. The digestive system is the body's lowest priority, when in a state of dehydration. The body will steal water from the bowels in the event it needs more elsewhere.

DAILY WATER CONSUMPTION CALCULATION

Children and adults should drink a minimum of half their body weight in ounces. For example: your child weighs 80 pounds. You will divide 80 in half to arrive at 40, then simple have them drink 40 ounces of water or more per day.

Many times, constipation is as simple as dehydration, even though you may not have been aware. Other times, while not the only source, proper hydration will provide relief along with a better diet.

Get them hydrated now! Make sure they have a water bottle or container that can be brought everywhere they go. Always remind them to take a drink, and to keep it on hand.

It takes roughly 4 weeks to rehydrate a child that has been dehydrated for a long period of time. Sippy cups of juice, soda pop, and milk are often confused as an equal substitute for water.

10 SIGNS OF DEHYDRATION

Pounding headache: The body desperately needs water and its sodium and potassium content. When dehydrated, a chemical reaction occurs in the blood triggering a headache.

Constipation: Water helps move food waste through the bowels and out of the body. If they are dehydrated their body has a hard time moving dry poo through the intestines, resulting in constipation and stomach pain.

Dizziness: One of the key signs of dehydration is when they quickly stand up and become very dizzy.

Cravings: When we are dehydrated, our body will crave sugars and carbohydrates.

Your Pee Is Extra Yellow: An obvious sign of dehydration is when their pee becomes a very dark shade of yellow. This means the urine is over-concentrated with waste and their body is limiting its water use in the digestive system.

Constant Fatigue: When they are dehydrated, blood pressure drops, reducing oxygen levels. This lack of oxygen slows our muscle and nerve functions, making us tired.

Overheating: Our body requires adequate water to regulate body temperature. When your child becomes dehydrated, it is rather easy for them to overheat and experience heat sensitivities.

Dry Mouth: An obvious indicator is a dry mouth and slightly swollen tongue. This is normally accompanied by bath breath.

Cramping: When dehydrated, our sodium and potassium stores become low and your child can end up with painful muscle spasms and general joint pain. This can be mistaken for growing pains, or Charlie horses.

Their Skin Isn't Bouncing Back: A simple test to see if they are dehydrated is the 'pinch test'. Pinch the skin on the back of the hand, and the tops of the finger joints to see how fast it bounces back. If it snaps back quickly, they are hydrated. However, if it is very slow then they are dehydrated. The back of the hand should bounce back instantly. While the fingers should take 1 second.

They Have Acne and Don't Know Why: Upper Zone Acne, which is the forehead, eyebrows, and temples are typically caused from internal dryness, digestion issues, and chronic dehydration. This can happen at any age, even as an infant.

4: Olive Oil Lemon Pow

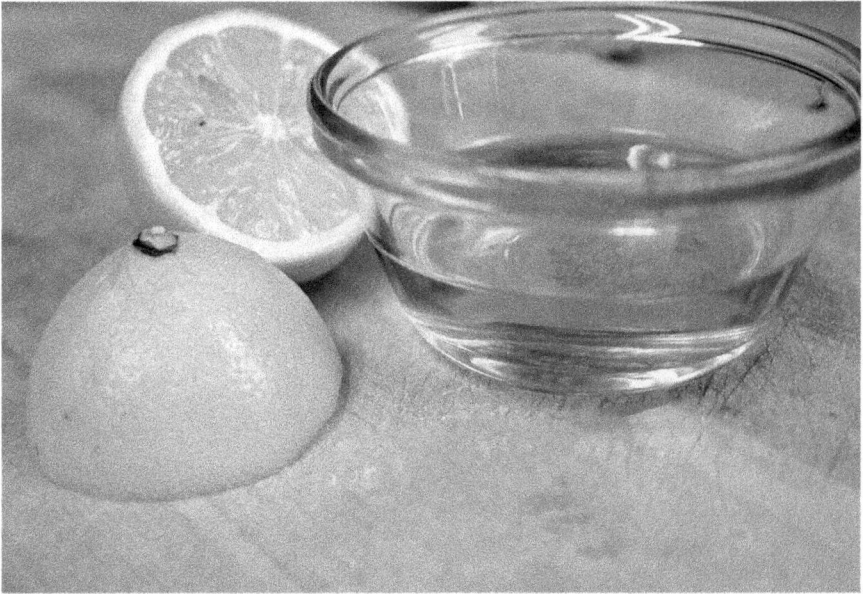

Pure olive oil can relieve constipation. It's not surprising based on its thick texture and consistency. It stimulates our digestive system, and helps move the poo through the colon with less pain and dryness. Taken daily can prevent constipation.

Ingredients:
- 1 tablespoon of olive oil
- 1 teaspoon of fresh squeezed lemon

DIRECTIONS
1. Upon waking in the morning take the olive oil and lemon mixture.
2. It works best on an empty stomach.

3. Can also take again 2-3 hours after lunch.

5: Warm Lemon Stimulant

The citric acid in lemon juice acts as a stimulant for our digestive system. It will flush out toxins and undigested material built-up. The warm water absorbs quickly into the colon for speedy results.

Ingredients:
- 1 fresh lemon
- 1 cup of warm water

DIRECTIONS
1. Squeeze one average sized lemon into 1 cup of warm water.
2. Drink first thing in the morning prior to eating.

6: Molasses Magic

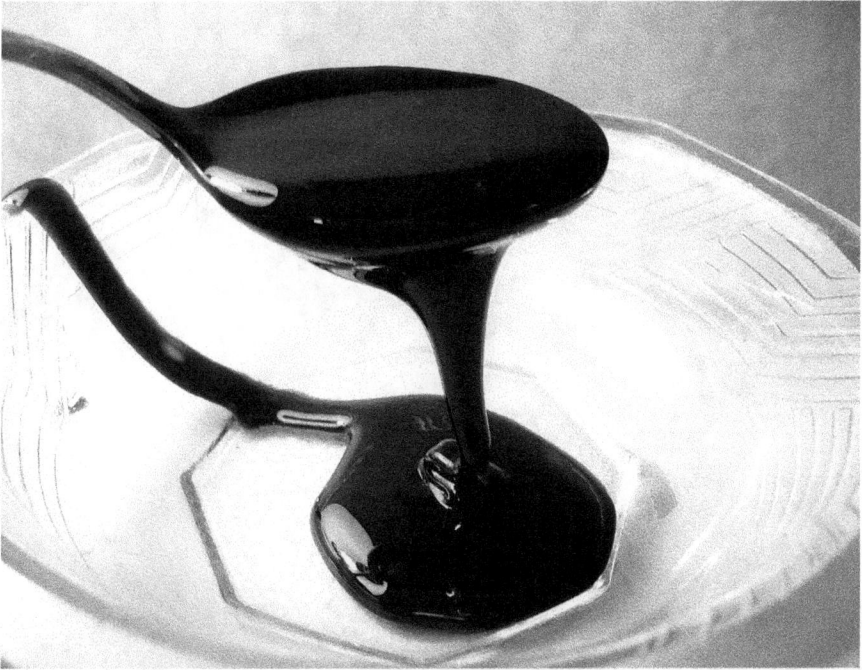

Blackstrap molasses contains a significant amount of vitamins and minerals, specifically magnesium. This is what relieves the constipation. It's natural, tasty, and works fast.

Ingredients:
- 1 teaspoon of blackstrap molasses
- 1 cup of warm water or unsweetened tea

DIRECTIONS
1. Add blackstrap molasses to warm water or tea.

2. Drink first thing in the morning on an empty stomach.

7: Brew A Coffee Poo

Caffeine is a natural stimulant for the digestive system. 1-2 cups are great, but too much can actually have the opposite effect. Coffee is a diuretic and makes you urinate more frequently. So, if consumed in excess, it can cause constipation by dehydrating the body and drawing out water that would normally soften our stool.

Coffee is a great stimulant for a younger teen who already enjoys a latte at their favorite coffee house. This is not intended for a small child.

DIRECTIONS
1. Drink one cup of coffee on an empty stomach first thing in the morning.
2. Having a small cup of coffee after lunch could also be beneficial.

8: Cardio Workout Kicks Constipation

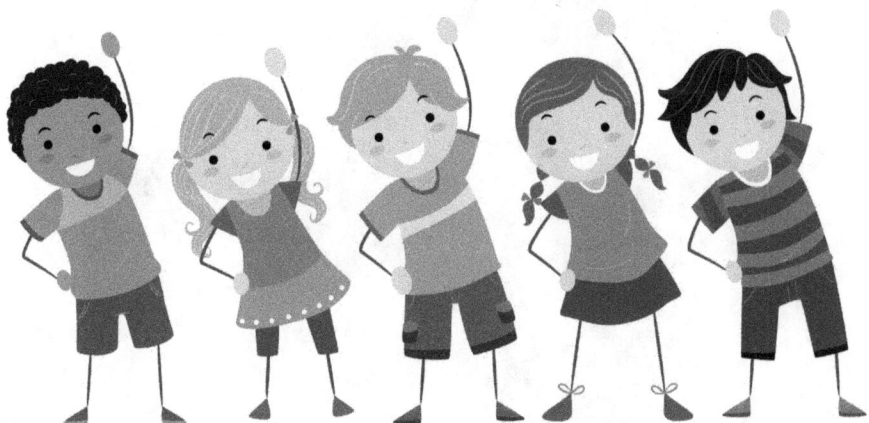

You may already know from experience that exercise can regulate bowels. More exercise equals more poop!

Exercise cuts down on the time it takes for food to pass through our large intestine. In turn, this limits the amount of water that gets absorbed from our stool into the body. The less water that the body takes from their stool, the softer your child's bowels become.

Exercise also speeds up their heart rate, which increases natural contractions of their intestinal muscles. So be sure to encourage them to get their heart rate up daily. This could mean going to the gym or doing some jump roping, hop scotch, jumping jacks, treadmill, playing catch, jogging or speed walking at your home.

9: Fantastic Fiber

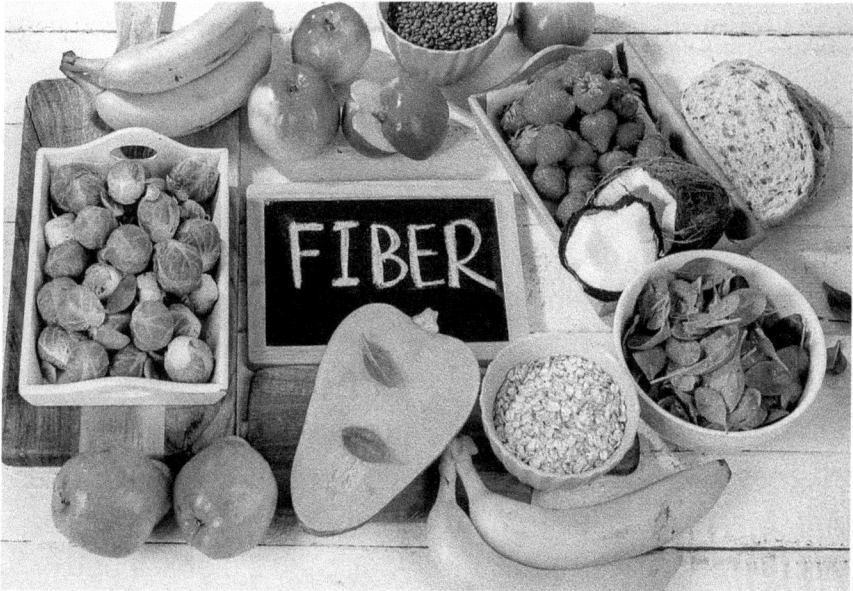

Our bodies know how to process fruits, veggies, grains and roughage more than refined or artificial foods. natural foods contain a plethora of fiber. Fiber is material that cannot be digested, and it acts like a sponge. It draws water from its surroundings, making it swell up, thus softening our poo.

SOME GOOD FIBER-FILLED FOODS INCLUDE:

LEGUMES

This group of veggies, which include beans, lentils, and peas, is full of health benefits. Include ½ cup of cooked legumes in your child's daily diet, which is around 15 grams of fiber. They are a rich source of fiber, as well as protein, vitamins, and minerals.

BROCCOLI

Add 1 cup of cooked broccoli for 5.5 grams of fiber.

OATMEAL

Oats are full of soluble fiber, which helps dissolve water from its surroundings, softening stool and making it easier for it to pass through the intestines. Include ½-1 cup of oatmeal in your child's daily diet.

SPINACH

1 cup of cooked spinach has 4 grams of fiber, and contains magnesium, a mineral that can really help you move that poo. Magnesium is often found in laxatives, but incorporating it naturally into your child's diet is a better long-term solution.

NUTS

Include ½ cup of nuts like pistachios, peanuts, almonds, or walnuts in their diet every day. They will provide them with almost 9 grams of fiber.

CHIA SEEDS OR FLAXSEEDS

Include two tablespoons of chia seeds or flaxseeds into your child's diet daily. They provide 5 grams of fiber.

BERRIES

½ cup of most berries will provide 4 grams of fiber.

PEARS

Pears are one of the most fibrous fruits, so adding them into their regular diet is a fantastic idea. One pear with the skin on, will provide almost 6 grams of fiber.

APPLES

A small apple with the skin on contains 3.6+ grams of fiber. The peels of many fruits contain insoluble fiber, which acts as a natural laxative.

PRUNES

Prunes are rich in fiber. ½ cup provides 6 grams of fiber and contains sorbitol and fructan, which are natural sugars that have a laxative effect.

RHUBARB

The senna and cascara compounds found in rhubarb can act as a natural laxative. Try incorporating rhubarb into a smoothing or make a laxative pie. If they are desperate to go poo, then rhubarb is an excellent choice!

ALOE

Like rhubarb, aloe also contains the same gut-flushing senna and cascara compounds.

ARTICHOKES

A cooked artichoke provides a whopping 10 grams of fiber.

GRAPES

Just 10 grapes provide 2.6 grams of fiber. Grapes can give some people diarrhea, which makes this a great snack for those with constipation.

10: Citrus-Flax Bowel Stimulator

Flaxseed oil coats the walls of the intestine, and increases the number of bowel movements they are having. When you add the flaxseed oil to a citrus loaded with fiber, you get the Citrus Flax Bowel Stimulator.

Ingredients:
- 1 glass of orange juice with pulp (8 oz.)
- 1 tablespoon of flaxseed oil

DIRECTIONS
1. Mix 1 tablespoon of flaxseed oil with 1 glass of orange juice.
2. Drink a glass every 5 hours.

11: Aloe Plant Intestinal Coat

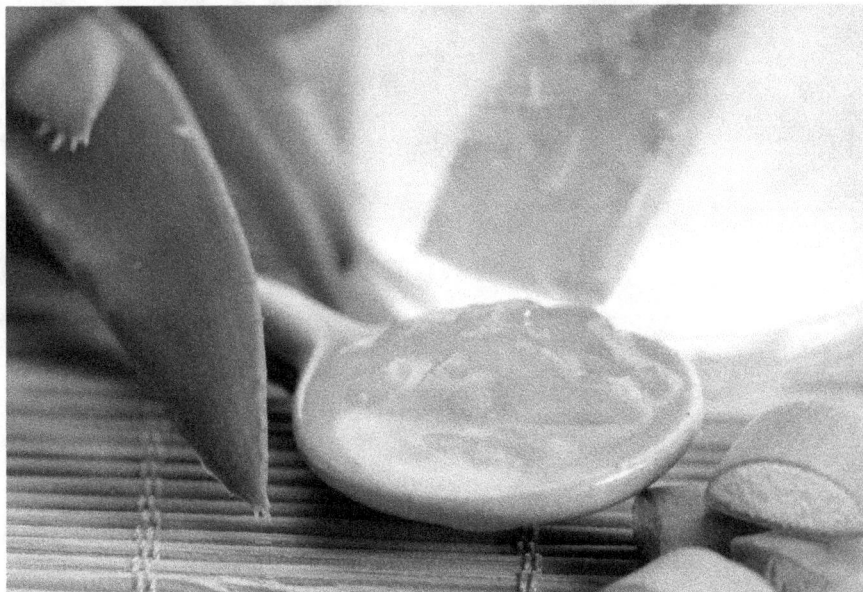

Aloe is known to soothe and coat the stomach and intestinal walls. It's best to use pure aloe vera gel from the plant. The gel straight from the plant is more concentrated.

Ingredients:
- 2 tablespoons of pure aloe gel
- 1 glass of orange juice with pulp 4-8 oz.

DIRECTIONS
1. Mix two tablespoons of pure gel with juice and drink in the morning.

12: Schedule A Poo

Potty schedules are not just for puppies or potty training toddlers. Regulating the timing of when older children go to the bathroom will regulate their bowel movements as well. Set aside about 15 minutes anywhere from 1-3 times a day, and try to go, even if nothing happens.

13: Baking Soda Explosion

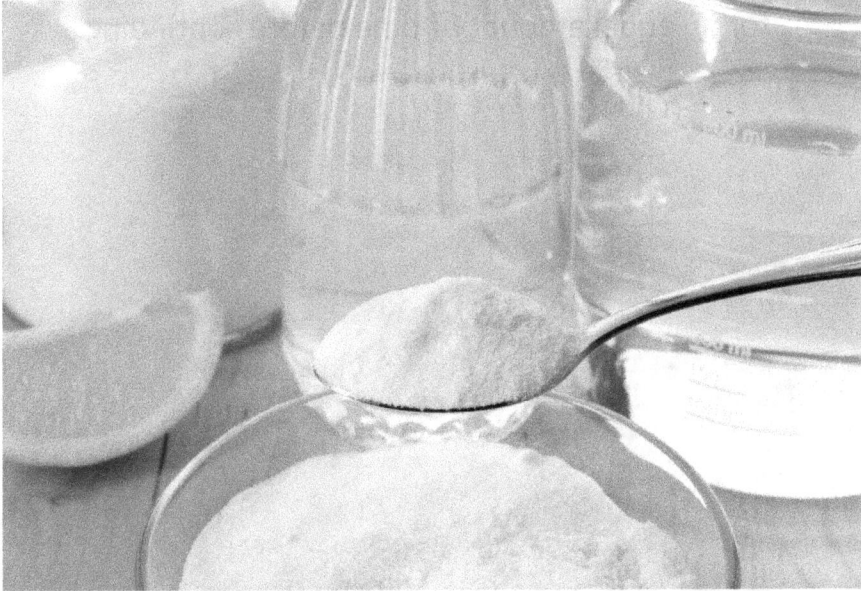

Baking soda works incredibly well for constipation. Because it is a bicarbonate, it will encourage air to come out of them one way or another. It also re-alkalizes the stomach, neutralizing the acid and helping things pass through the gut.

Ingredients:
- ¼ teaspoon baking soda
- 1/4 cup warm water

DIRECTIONS
2.   Mix a ¼ teaspoon of baking soda with ¼ cup of warm water. You can go up to ½ teaspoon for children over 80lbs.

3. Drink quickly.
4. Consume once daily for up to 3-4 days, then refrain for an equal amount of time before continuing.

14: Epsom Salt Stool Softener

Epsom salt draws water from its surroundings, softening up stool and makes it easy to pass. Magnesium also promotes contraction of the bowel muscles.

Ingredients:
- 1/2 teaspoons of Epsom salt
- 1 cup of water or 100% fruit juice or cold pressed juice

DIRECTIONS
1. Dissolve 1/2 teaspoons of Epsom salt in one cup of water.
2. Drink every 4 hours as needed.

15: Magnesium Madness

Magnesium can dramatically improve constipation.

DIRECTIONS

- Consume about 100-125 milligrams 2x daily.
- Cut back on milligrams if they are having diarrhea.

16: Jolly Prune Juice

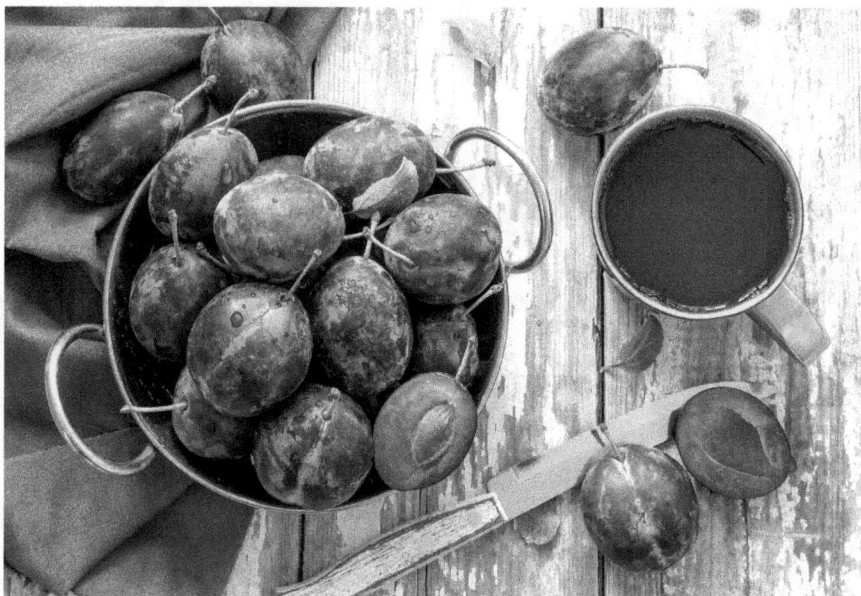

This is a classic cure for constipation. The fruit works as a natural laxative because of its high fiber, and sorbitol content. Sorbitol causes poo to draw water from its surroundings, providing them with a soft stool that is easy to pass.

Ingredients:
- 1 glass of prune juice (8oz)

DIRECTIONS
1. Drink one glass of prune juice in the morning and one at night.

17: Daily Prune Program

Prunes are incredible at relieving constipation. They are filled with soluble fiber which slows digestion and aids nutrient absorption. Prunes also contain insoluble fiber which bulks up the stool, making it pass more quickly through our intestines. Prunes have an abundant of sorbitol, which increases water levels in the stool.

DIRECTIONS

1. Eat 2-6 whole prunes every day.
2. You can also chop them up and add to your child's oatmeal and/or to a smoothie.
3. Whole prunes will need to have the pit removed before consumption.

18: Get Going with Ginger

Ginger is a powerful laxative and has so many wonderful health benefits.

Ingredients:
- 1/8 teaspoon of fresh grated ginger
- 1 cup of water/or tea

DIRECTIONS
1. Add fresh grated ginger in 1 cup of warm water or tea.
2. Drink 1-2 times daily and increase ginger for a stronger effect.
3. Go slow if you choose to add more ginger, it can make them feel a bit jittery.

19: Free Your Bowels with Fennel

Fennel is commonly used to facilitate a proper poo. It stimulates the secretion of digestive and gastric juices while soothing inflammation in the stomach. It also reduces flatulence. Fennel is best used in its whole form for constipation to benefit from the whole seed.

Ingredients:
- ½ teaspoon of dried fennel seeds
- 1 cup of water

DIRECTIONS
1. Crush the fennel seeds into a course powder.
2. Add to a tea bag, or tea cloth.
3. Heat 1 cup of water to a hot temperature (do not bring to a boil).
4. Pour hot water over fennel, cover and let rest for 10 minutes. Let cool.
5. Drink up to 3 times a daily, after meals.

20: Identifying Weak Peristaltic Signals

This method is very straightforward, but is often ignored in our daily lives. When your child feels the need to go to the bathroom, they must go immediately. For kids with chronic constipation, this may be one of the most important pieces of advice. Our body is giving us the signal for a reason, and you must listen. The longer you hold it, the more water is absorbed from the stool, and the harder and dryer it becomes.

Our body will only send signal to have a bowel movement for a certain amount of time. After that, the contraction begins to decline, and the feeling goes away. This is how we begin the cycle of constipation.

As you are helping your child change their diet and incorporating poo-approved foods, water and probiotics, watching for the first sign of a peristaltic signal is the key.

21: Chia and Flaxseed Oil Colon Food

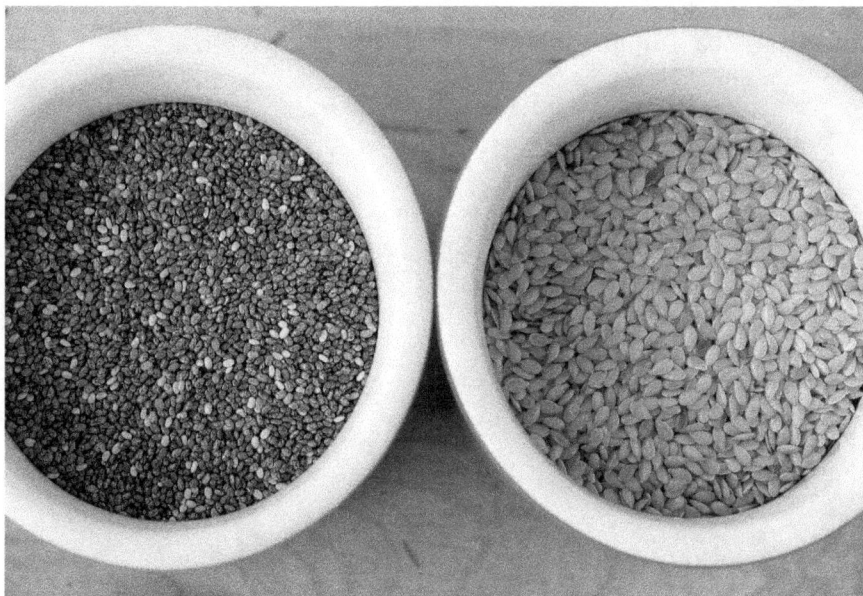

Sprouted chia seeds and flaxseeds are high in fiber and healthy fats. Flaxseed oil does an excellent job at lubricating the colon.

You may need to be sneaky at adding these two ingredients into your child's diet. Chia seeds are fun in juices, because of their unique texture. While flaxseed oil can be added to a fruit smoothie, or salad dressing without too much notice.

DIRECTIONS: Chia Seeds

- Take 1-2 tablespoons of pre-soaked chia seeds daily with water.

DIRECTIONS: <u>Flaxseed oil</u>

- Take 1/2 tablespoon of flaxseed oil daily.

22: Psyllium Husk Poo Paradise

Psyllium husk is super high in fiber and helpful for forming a good poo. When combined with water, psyllium husk swells, which stimulates the intestines to contract.

DIRECTIONS

1.   Mix 1/2 tablespoon with 8 ounces of juice.
2.   Consume 1 time per day.

23: Cod Liver Oil & Carrot Elixir

Cod liver oil is an old remedy that has been successfully helping constipation sufferers. You can normally find the fresh pressed carrot juice at your local natural grocery store, or do it yourself with a juicer.

Ingredients:

- 1/2 tablespoon of cod liver oil
- 4 ounces of fresh pressed carrot juice

DIRECTIONS

1. Take 1/2 tablespoon of cod liver oil with 4 ounces of fresh pressed carrot juice.
2. Can be taken up to 2 times daily.

24: Apple Fiber Blast

Apple fiber contain a substance called pectin. Pectin is insoluble fiber that helps the stool become bulky, forcing the intestines to contract.

DIRECTIONS
- Consume 1 teaspoons of apple fiber 2 times daily.

25: Dandelion Doo-Doo Tea

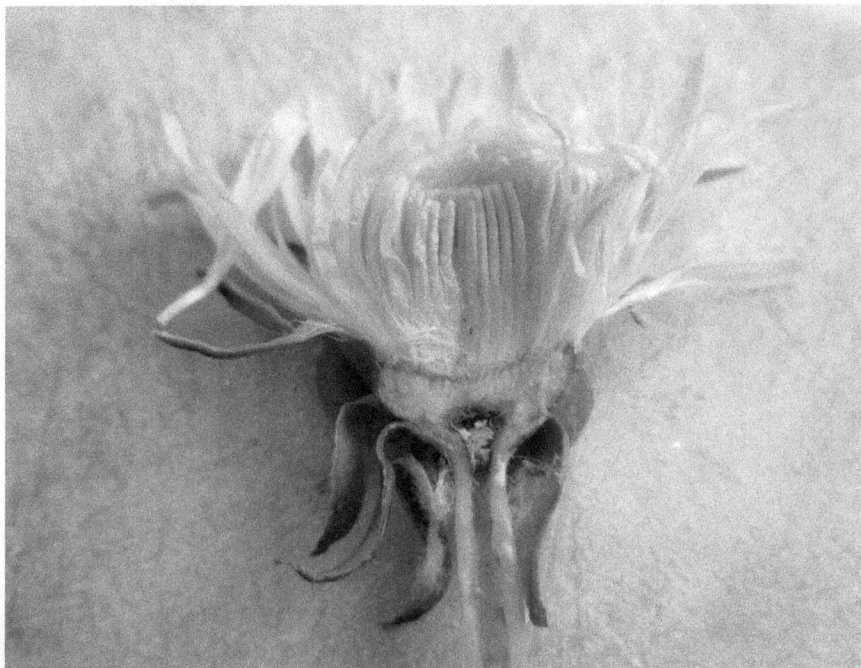

Dandelions are tremendous for relieving constipation. They are considered a gentle laxative as well as a detoxifier.

Ingredients:
- 1 teaspoons of dried dandelion leaves
- 1 cup of hot water

DIRECTIONS
1. Place 1 teaspoons of dried dandelion leaves in a tea bag.
2. Pour hot water over them.

3. Cover and let steep for 6-10 minutes. Let cool.
4. Drink up to 3 times daily.

26: Yummy Yogurt

yogurt is filled with probiotics and can increase your child's good gut bacteria. Be careful about eating to many dairy products, they can slow down our digestive system in large quantities. If your child is allergic to dairy, then stick with the probiotic supplements only.

DIRECTIONS
- Eat ½-1 cup of high quality yogurt daily and or enjoy it in a smoothie.

27: Poop Stool

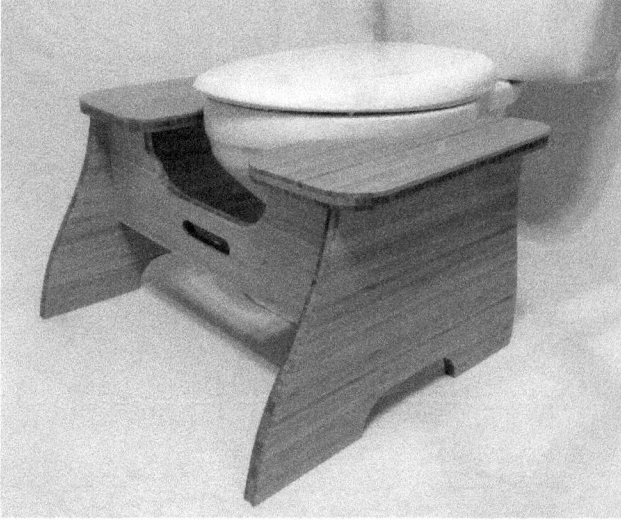

Using a poop stool when sitting on the toilet forces you to open your colon much like you would in nature. Pooping in the natural squat position makes pooping faster, more complete, and reduces straining of your entire body.

Squatting rather than sitting could help prevent things like constipation, appendicitis, hemorrhoids, colon cancer, IBS, hernias, diverticulosis, and pelvic organ prolapse.

28: Colon Detox

The best thing you can do for the health of the colon is a semi-annual colon cleanse and detox. It will remove old fecal matter and waste from the colon, heavy metals and drug residues. It will also strengthen the colon muscle, repair any damage, and eliminates polyps and other abnormal growths. It's an excellent way to maintain good gut health and avoid future constipation.

Start your child off with a simple and gentle colon detox. Follow the manufactures age and weight instructions for a proper dosage.

29: Colon Hydrotherapy

Colon hydrotherapy is an excellent way to kickstart their constipation free life. The idea of colon hydrotherapy or colonics makes some people a little squeamish or even embarrassed, but it is well worth a try. The process is very simple and has been used since ancient times to rid the body of sickness.

Hard dry poo that is backing you up is made of impacted feces, dead cellular tissue, accumulated mucous, parasites, and worms. This is very poisonous to our body because the toxins re-enter and circulate in the blood stream. It impairs the colon's ability to absorb vitamins and minerals. And finally, it causes sluggish bowel movements and terrible constipation. Colon Hydrotherapy or colonics works at removing the impacted feces after constipation has already set in.

If your child has been suffering from chronic constipation, then it would be a great idea to find a professional colon hydro-therapist in your area to discuss.

30: Oil Lubes the Tubes

Constipated individuals always benefit from consuming raw, unrefined oils. Besides the high nutrition value, oil is excellent for coating the intestines and helping pass hard dry poo. It is important to consume oil daily for constant intestinal support.

Best Raw Unrefined Oils

COCONUT OIL: Coconut oil contains medium-chain fatty acids that are easily digested and utilized as an energy burning fuel, instead of being stored as fat.

Coconut oil is high in good-saturated fats, along with lauric acid, which our body converts to monolaurin. Monolaurin is a natural antiviral agent that aids our body in eliminating parasites, viruses, bacteria, yeast and fungi.

Directions
- Consume 1 tablespoon of coconut oil daily.

OLIVE OIL: Olive oil is the oil extracted from the olive fruit. A popular oil known to be a heart healthy monounsaturated fat high in oleic acid. Olive oil is also composed of palmitic acid, linoleic acid, stearic acid and small amounts of alpha-linolenic acid.

The best olive oil to use is raw unrefined extra virgin olive oil, which is typically a golden-green color.

Directions
- Consume 1/2 tablespoon of olive oil daily.

RED PALM OIL: Red palm oil comes from palm fruit, and is composed of palmitic, stearic, oleic and linoleic acids.

Like coconut oil, its plant base saturated fats are made up of "medium chain fatty acids." These are "good fats" to consume because they increase metabolism and are easily digested, providing an instant energy source. Red palm oil gets its super rich orange-red color from the presence of carotenes.

Directions
- Consume 1/2 tablespoon of red palm oil daily.

HEMP SEED OIL: Hemp seed oil is another type of good fat pressed from the seeds of the hemp plant. Consuming hemp oil is incredible for our digestive system, as it nourishes cell membranes and provides antifungal, antibacterial and antiviral properties. It is also high in the antioxidants vitamin E and beta-carotene and also includes the rare gamma-linolenic acid (GLA) and stearidonic acid (SDA).

Quality hemp seed oil is unrefined, cold pressed, always dark in color and preferably preserved in dark glass bottles.

Directions

- Consume 1/2 tablespoon of the oil daily.

31: Dairy Products Clogs the Derriere

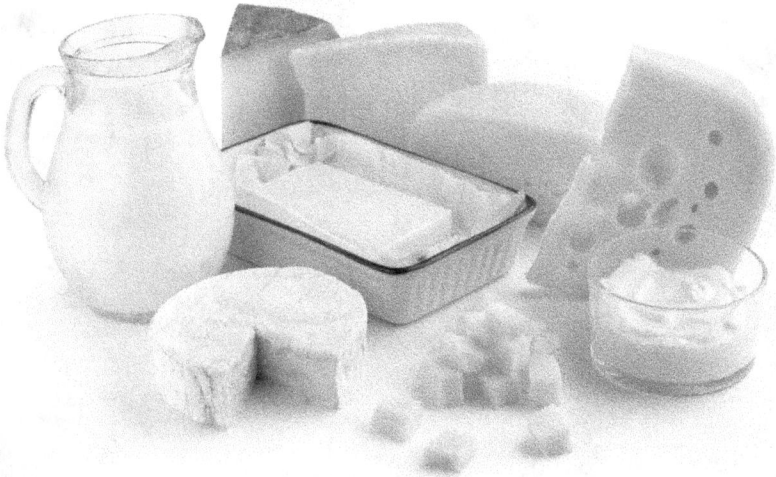

Since dairy is processed very slow in our bodies, fatty dairy products may cause or worsen constipation. Dairy also contains lactose, which causes painful gas and bloating. For many people that consume an enormous amount of dairy products, cutting it out for two full weeks could be an excellent choice to give your gut a break.

When reintroducing it back into their diet, go slow and monitor its effects.

32: Foods That Can Cause Diarrhea

If you are looking for a natural way to get the poo moving faster, try packing your child's meals full of foods that are known to cause diarrhea.

FRUITS INCLUDE:
- pears
- apples
- most berries
- figs
- prunes
- dates
- raisins
-

HIGH-FIBER VEGETABLES INCLUDE:
- broccoli
- Brussels sprouts
- cabbage
- carrots
- artichokes
- peas

33: Figs for The Fanny

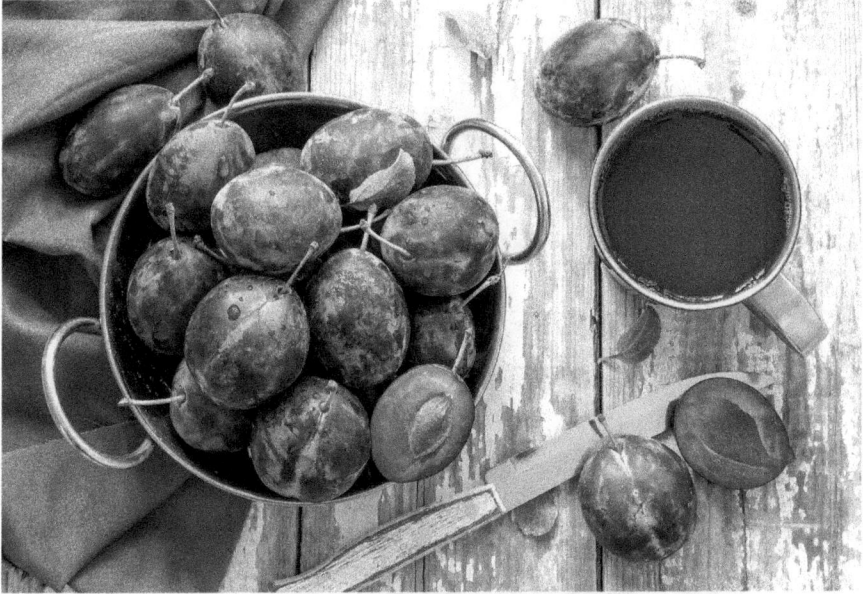

Figs are small, wrinkled-looking fruits that belong to the mulberry family. Although you can eat figs fresh off the vine, most people prefer dried figs. Figs contain fiber that can have health benefits for your child's gastrointestinal tract. They taste great diced up and added for a sweet touch in cereals, trail mix, cookies or smoothies.

DIRECTIONS
- Consume 2-4 figs daily (whole or chopped).
- Increase daily if desired.

34: Hot Honey Tush Push Drink

This is an excellent way to force the body to produce a bowel movement. Drink this honey, ginger and fennel beverage first thing in the morning.

Ingredients:
- 2 teaspoons raw honey
- 1 drop ginger essential oils (food grade)
- 1 drop fennel essential oils (food grade)
- 1 glass of hot water

DIRECTIONS
1. Boil water and mix in your ingredients
2. Let it cool until they can safely drink.

35: Move the Poo: Abdominal Massage Lotion

By massaging your child's stomach, you are capable of helping the poo move through the intestines. Do not rub hard, but a nice gentle massage is known to produce a poo the following morning. The essential oils used also aid in the stimulation of the colon.

Ingredients:
- 2 drops peppermint essential oils
- 1 drop black pepper essential oils
- 1 tsp warmed grapeseed or sweet almond oil

DIRECTIONS
1. Combine ingredients in a small non-reactive bowl.
2. Massage blend over abdomen in a clockwise direction.
3. Repeat 2 to 3 times daily or as desired.
4. Use the alternative oils below if needed.

Alternative Essential Oils:
- Fennel
- Ginger
- Petitgrain
- Rosemary
- Spearmint
- Basil
- Peppermint

36: Rump Reliever: Circulation Boosting Massage Oil

This massage oil will relax the colon, intestines and aid in proper digestion of food. It will improve circulation and boost their bodies detoxification process.

Ingredients:
- 6 drops of rosemary or neroli essential oils
- 6 drops fennel essential oils
- 2 ounces carrier oil (coconut, sweet almond, or jojoba)

DIRECTIONS
1. Combine carrier oil and essential oils in a bowl or 2 oz. glass container.
2. Apply this oil to the abdomen and lower back, a little goes a long way.
3. Use 1-2 daily.

37: Bum Bath: Essential Oil Infused Bath

An easy way to help get your child's digestion flowing, is to take a warm bath with digestive supporting essential oils.

Ingredients:
- 1 cups Epsom salts
- 1/4 cup baking soda
- 1/8 cup sea salt
- 10 drops essential oils

DIRECTIONS
1. Add all ingredients together in a container.
2. Stir into a warm bath.
3. Choose your favorite oil from the list below.

Colon Supporting Essential Oils
- Carrot seed
- Celery seed
- Juniper
- Dill
- Grapefruit
- Tangerine
- Lime
- Palmarosa
- Lemon

38: Juicing

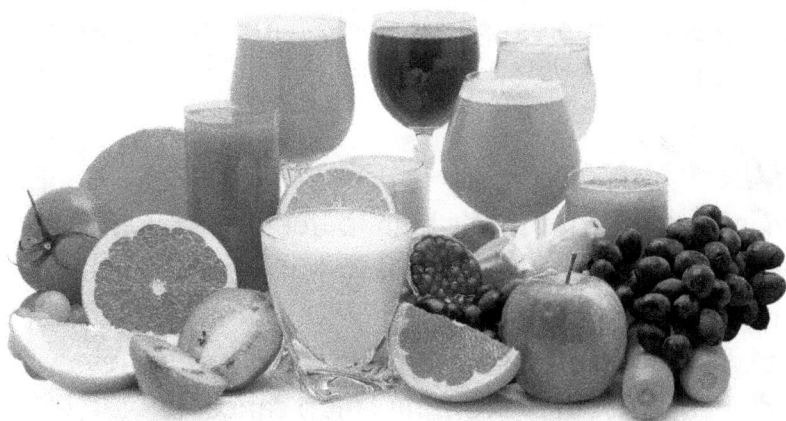

Juicing is a quick and natural way to get their blocked system moving quickly. Juicing forces your child to eat/drink large amounts of fruits and vegetables that provide their body with fiber. Fiber bulks our stool and helps soft, moist poo move through the intestines effortlessly.

There are certain fruits and vegetables that do the best job when it comes to constipation. When choosing fruits and veggies for constipation, look for options that are high in fiber and low in sugar.

Find recipes that include both fruits and veggies for the best flavors your child will enjoy.

APPLES

Apples contain flavonoids, phytonutrients and other vitamins and minerals that are extremely beneficial to the body. They're a very popular fruit when it comes to aiding our digestion. Apples can also help with heart disease and the regulation of blood fat levels.

KIWI

Kiwi is another fruit that's high in fiber and low in sugar. Kiwi is loaded with vitamin C, K, and E, copper, fiber, manganese, copper, folate and potassium. This incredible fruit will help to bind and remove toxins from their colon, which can assist in preventing colon cancer later in life.

ORANGES

Oranges are well-known for their high dose of vitamin C and immune-boosting powers. However, oranges also contain flavonoids that aids in the relief of constipation. It has been found that oranges play the role of a natural, completely safe, and long-term laxative.

SPINACH

When it comes to constipation, eating spinach is very important. The Magnesium in spinach can actually help the colon contract and attract water to help better flush things through.

BEETS

Beets are great to juice when you are constipated. They provide a handful of colon supporting fibers, vitamins and minerals. However, there is something much more interesting about beets that you are probably not aware of.

Beat Test

Beets are known for being a safe way to test patient bowl movements. By using the "beet test" you can figure out if you are eliminating within the preferred 12-24-hour range.

How do you do a beet test? You simply eat some beets and then wait until your child poops. If you see a fiery red bowel movement in 24 hours or less, then they are digesting well. If it takes more than 24 hours for the red bowel movements to appear then they have a "slow transit time" which can be helped by increasing thier fiber and water intake.

Make sure that when fiber is increased that water is also increased.

Beet-Sweet Juice Blend

Use a juicer for these recipes. Blend together and drink.

Ingredients:
- 3 small beets
- 2 green apples
- 2 carrots

- 1 cup of raw fresh spinach
- 1 tablespoon of chia or flaxseed oil

Apple-Kiwi Juice Blend

Use a juicer for these recipes. Blend together and drink.

Ingredients:
- 3 ½ kiwis (peeled)
- 2 green apples
- 1 cup of raw fresh spinach
- ½ lemon peeled

Green-Citrus Juice Blend

Use a juicer for these recipes. Blend together and drink.

Ingredients:
- 2 oranges
- 2 ½ green apples
- 2 cups of raw fresh spinach

39: Raw Food Diet

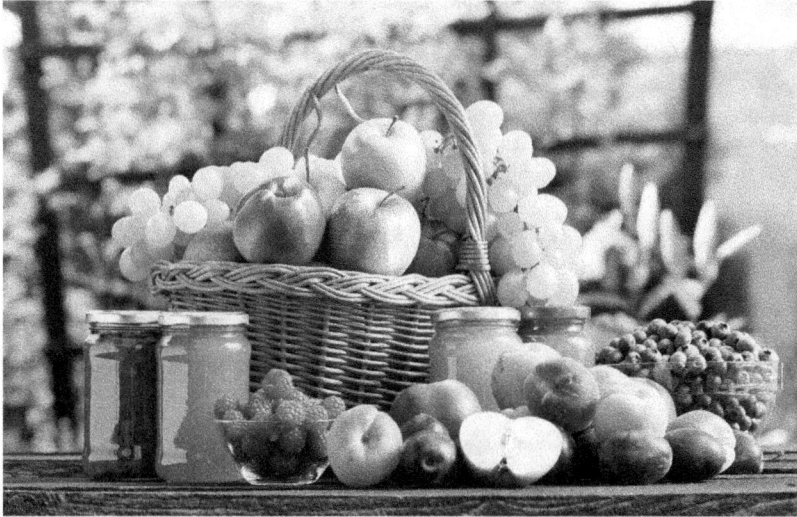

If you slowly begin incorporating raw foods into your child's diet, you will be amazed at their increased energy levels, regular bowl movements, and ability to focus. A raw food diet is essentially providing the body with all the fiber, nutrition and hydration it needs to run at optimal levels.

ADDITIONAL BENEFITS

Additional benefits include, improved skin appearance and fullness, weight loss, improved digestion, and the reduction of many diseases such as heart disease, diabetes, and cancer, both now and the future.

40: Bone Broth for the Booty

Bone Broth Heals Your Gut! One of the most vital nutrients for healing the gut and intestinal track is gelatin. This substance is found in abundance in bone broth.

The intestinal lining is supposed to be permeable for nutrients to pass through. However, this lining can become too permeable due to lifestyle factors such as poor diet, dehydration, stress, as well as bacterial and fungal overgrowths.

It is much like poking huge holes in your window screens at home. Yes, the good air will pass through, but the flies, gnats, and mosquitoes will too. Undigested food particles can slip through the gut lining and pass directly into the bloodstream. When this happens, the immune system starts attacking the very foods your child eats, we typically call these food sensitivities.

Why will the gelatin in bone broth heal your child's gut?
- The gelatin in bone broth spackles the excess holes in the gut lining.
- It also soothes the digestive track including reducing the inflammation in the bowels.
- In addition, the gelatin provides a more slippery surface area inside the intestines.
- The gel allows poop to easily move through.
- Drink one cup or bowl of bone broth soup daily.

41: Remove Food Allergens

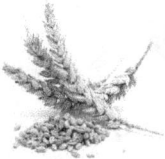
Gluten & Wheat

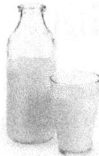
Cow's Milk

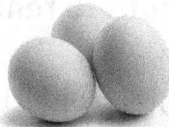
Eggs

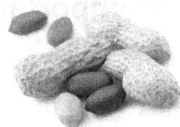
Peanuts

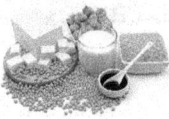
Soy Products

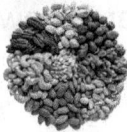
Tree Nuts

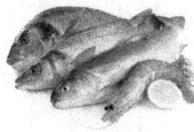
Seafood

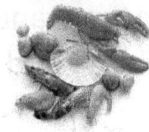
Shellfish

Removing food allergens from your child's diet may be the last item on the list, but not the least important by any means. Food allergies typically trigger an autoimmune response, thus causing our bodies to experience chronic inflammation.

Long-term chronic inflammation effects our intestines and digestive system, leads to more severe diseases later in life. If you have tried everything, removing the top major food allergens from your child's diets is essential.

The group of the eight major allergenic foods comprise of milk, eggs, fish, crustacean shellfish, tree nuts, peanuts, wheat and soybean.

These foods account for about 90% of all food allergies in the United States and must be declared on any processed food by law.

Most important foods to remove right now:

- You should start with dairy and wheat products.

Diary and wheat products are hard for our bodies to consume and break down. They are known to cause children and adults serious constipation.

After the removal of these two food groups, give your child up to two weeks before removing another one of the eight allergens on the list if necessary.

You have removed all eight allergens, hydrated, increased fiber and nothing is working, remove Nightshades.

Nightshades seem harmless; however, they are also inflammatory foods if consumed regularly.

Some of the most popular nightshades are potatoes, tomatoes, bell peppers, and chili peppers. But because various spices and spice mixes are made from chili peppers, nightshades can be found in a whole host of processed foods!

What nightshades you should remove now:
- Regular potatoes, tomatoes and bell peppers.

This does not include sweet potato varieties, since they are not from the same family as regular potatoes. You are free to replace all of your child's potato consumption with those sweet potato or yam varieties.

Where to Begin

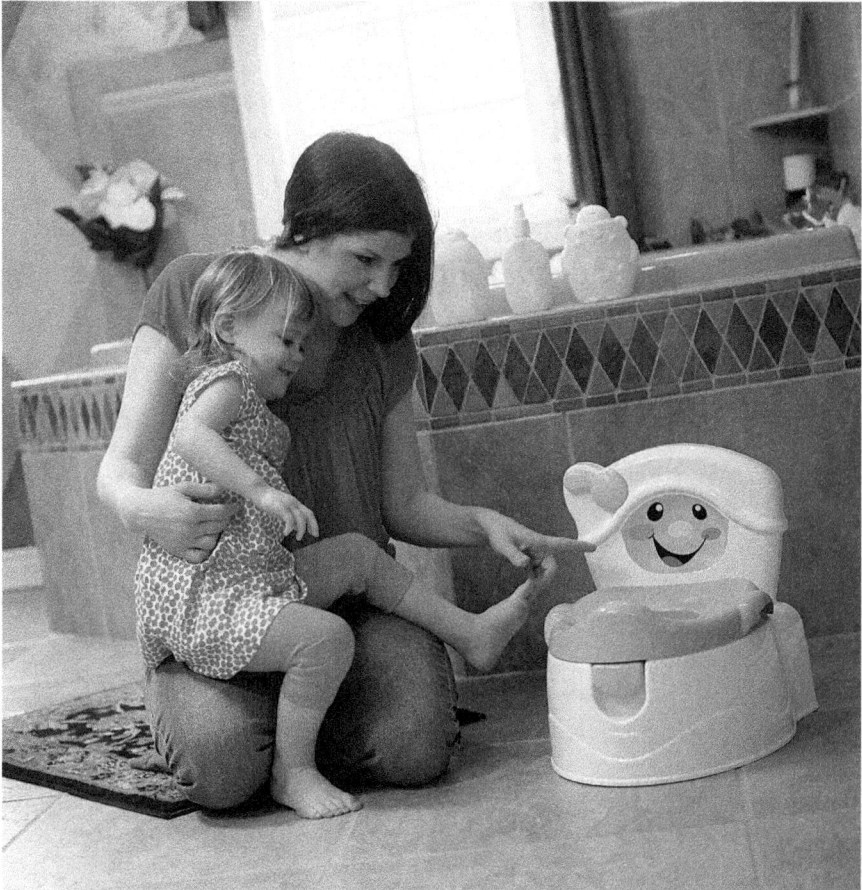

There is no right or wrong, or one size fits all when it comes to our individual bodies. But there are general ways to approach this health issue and achieve success, if you are willing to change current habits.

Here are the steps that everyone should take to begin the journey of a life free of constipation. As you follow along, be sure to add many, or all the suggested items 1-39 in this book.

DAILY RECOMMENDATION:

1. Start By purchasing a high-quality probiotic. At least 15 billion and raw for daily consumption. These probiotics can be a little expensive, but they are worth every penny if your child is a constant sufferer of constipation. Most stores will carry a chewable for children, or they can be easily ordered online.

2. Get a poop stool to go to the bathroom without strain. If you cannot find one and need it now, anything sturdy to get their knees in an upward position would be a good substitute. It's very difficult to poo when your feet are dangling above the toilet.

3. Start today by serving fresh fruits and lightly cooked vegetable, or salads, as the staple of all your meals. You could include a very small portion of meat. Getting fiber is a must to overcome hard, slow poo. Fruits and vegetables have a high-water content to help with dehydration. They are good food for the new probiotics to eat and flourish.

4. Take one of the oils listed in Chapter 30: Oil Lubes the Tubes daily.

5. Have them care a water bottle always, and sip once every 5 to 10 minutes or more. Be sure to have them drink at least half their body weight in ounces or more daily. This is a vital component to living constipation free – water-water-water!

   FYI: 90% of all patients can be cured of constipation by just drinking the correct amount of water, with only little changes to their overall diet.

6. Only drink 1 cup of coffee, tea or other caffeinated beverages daily. They cause our body to dump liquids, and that is not helpful when we are trying to hydrate.

7. Eat a bowl of oatmeal daily. This is an easy way to bulk up the stool with little effort, and most children can enjoy the flavor.

8. Get your child to attempt to poo after every meal. Also, remind them to carefully feel for the peristaltic waves, and get to the restroom immediately. DO NOT DELAY!

9. If you have tried everything, then begin removing the top 8 allergen foods, common nightshades and add bone broth to their diet.

- Focus on using one or more tricks per day, until you find a few things that really get their poo to move. Continue using them as an excellent way to maintain a healthy gut and relieve the devastating effects of chronic or occasional constipation.

www.ingramcontent.com/pod-product-compliance
Lightning Source LLC
Chambersburg PA
CBHW050534280326
41933CB00011B/1583